I0438814

My Wine Diet

How Losing Weight & Drinking Wine Changed My Life

Copyright © 2014 Jackie Clark.

ISBN-13:978-1494998462

ISBN-10:1494998467

This book is the story of how I lost weight and achieved the weight I wanted to be. I have taken control of my weight for the first time in my life.

I must stress that:

- I am not medically trained.
- I am not a nutritionist.
- I am not a professional in any of these disciplines.
- I did join a gym part way through the six months.

I have, however, over the years tried dozens of diets and have learned what does and doesn't work for me.

This is my story, including what I ate during six months of my life. I have felt healthy and believe I am eating well. Should anyone who reads this book wish to follow the diet I follow, they must consult an expert such as a doctor or dietician before doing so.

This diet method suits me. It may not suit anyone else and may or may not be suitable for others to follow.

The reader of this book is solely responsible, for ascertaining if this type of eating plan is suitable for them. The actual food choices in the day by day listing suited me. The choices may not be suitable for anyone else.

Consult a doctor or other professional before embarking on this type of eating plan.

I did not start out to write a book on dieting. I did not intend to write a book at all. I do write recipe and music books but writing this book was not my intention

It came about by accident. January 2012 arrived with me as usual the wrong weight. Christmas always does this to me. To be honest I over eat and drink at Christmas. Most of us do, and then frantically attempt to lose it quickly before returning to work. This approach never worked for me and I suspect not for others either.

So I am 30 pounds or so overweight and need to lose it. I have tried dozens of diets over the years and joined every slimming club I could find with varying results.

The problem I found with all diets is the starting point. I reduce my food intake and lose no weight; I reduce more and lose no weight. Eventually I begin to lose weight. There is a tipping point at which I begin to lose weight. The problem is, that by the time I have found that point, I am bored, and decided that the diet is too slow, and I have probably taken my food intake too low and am starving hungry. Of course, my other issue is putting weight back on again at the end of the diet.

I have learned over the years what my body responds to and decided on a food level that I suspected was right for me. It was a suitable point to start, and within a short time, I lost weight, and, spurred on by my success in the first few weeks I carried on losing weight and was happy with my food intake.

So accidentally I found the starting point. Perhaps I sub consciously used the experience of past diets, who knows. Having lost the few pounds I wanted to lose. I thought I would continue and try to lose as many of the 30 pounds; I needed to lose as I could. I did not want to be hungry or give up wine or other goodies so I thought I would continue eating as I was. I had lost my few pounds easily and drank wine throughout.

I do know that two things have helped me above all others in the past when losing weight. Writing everything down that I eat (this really is not a chore, a little like writing a shopping list, but after you have bought the shopping.) The second thing is weighing food. I have found that by trying to use volume I am out by large amounts. Try pouring two identical amounts of a light breakfast cereal into two similar sized dishes. Then weigh them and see the difference, this experiment amazed me.

I am tired of diets taking over my life and food ruling me. I love food, the textures, the tastes, the temperature differences. I write recipe books so I am always testing and trying foods. Food is not my enemy. I enjoy it and do not want to be frightened to eat. I also like my wine in the evening. I decided that if I am to enjoy my food, enjoy my wine and enjoy eating out I needed to forget dieting and choose a way of eating that allowed for:

- The pleasures of eating lovely food.
- The pleasure of wine.
- Be able to eat out without feeling guilt.
- Lose weight.

- Be able to adjust my diet to maintain my weight, once my target weight was achieved.

More importantly I intended to be totally in control of my weight, and not my weight in control of me.

Did I achieve these goals? Yes, I did. I then decided to share my results.

This is not a diet book as such, it is a method of taking control of eating that allows me to reduce or increase my weight as I choose. This is a story of my journey that took just over six months and allows me to eat almost everything I want, enjoy my wine and eat out when I want.

When the pounds go on, I know what to adjust to lose them again. A one-night spree may put a few pounds on that will take a week or so to lose, but I don't worry about it because during my six-month journey, I learned what works for me and what does not. I did increase my exercise levels part way through the diet by joining a gym. The diet is not totally responsible for all my loss although initially, the gym had no effect, I suspect it did later.

Essentially I realised that the diets followed and slimming clubs joined have left me floundering. I lost weight but had no idea how, other than the obvious eating less. I did not know the point at which my weight balanced with my food. Knowing my tipping point allows me to be in complete control. Without knowing where my tipping or balancing point is. Dieting and slimming clubs left me in limbo. Now I am in complete control.

My story started a few days after Christmas 2012. I reduced my food intake by a small amount to lose a few pounds that I had put on over Christmas. I did not write anything down at this point. After the first week, my weight had dropped by 1.25 pounds. Now I did not cut down by much; I still drank my wine and had other goodies. I realized that I was enjoying my food and losing weight even after having treated myself. I decided that if I could lose weight by doing what I was doing. Instead of being a martyr to yet another oddball diet, I could continue this way, lose weight and enjoy this way of eating long term. I also really needed to lose more than a few pounds. Rather a lot of pounds needed to be removed from my body.

I decided that I would attempt to use this method of eating as a lifestyle choice. I would not drink gallons of wine or eat pounds of chocolate, but I was not going to give them up. My intention was once and for all to take control of my weight, eat goodies, drink wine and not shy away from going out for meals, etc. I could, have done as I had in the past. That is to go on a crash diet, lose the weight and then go back to normal eating and put weight on again. I was utterly sick to death of doing that. My whole life, was dieting to lose weight.

I wrote down what I remembered I had eaten during the previous week, so I could know my starting point. Over the following months, I kept records of my food intake. I had good weeks and bad weeks and adjusted my food to suit my weight loss or lack of it. As my weight reduced, I reduced my food intake as I needed less energy to carry me about, so needed less food. Sometimes I got it incorrect and felt a little hungry so had to adjust accordingly. Often I got it wrong and gained weight.

Over the months, my weight slowly reduced, and I learned what worked for me. One thing I did learn was to not be in a hurry. If my weight loss slowed I did not reduce my food intake by a significant amount. I reduced it slightly and then waited a few days to see the result. I usually waited a week. What I eat today will not affect my weight tomorrow. My weight changes days after eating a lot extra or cutting out a lot of food.

I reduced my food intake by reducing quantities slightly, an ounce, less meat or a smaller slice of bread or even 5 gram off my cereal allowance, according to the amount of weight I lost or didn't. By around day 166, I had a problem with losing weight. I seemed to have gone into free fall, after achieving my target weight. I did not want to eat junk food to stop weight loss or increase my food intake dramatically as that would ruin my control. I increased my food slightly each week until my weight did stop reducing. I was then able to stay in control by changing my food intake by very small amounts. I did not attempt to increase exercise levels to control my weight, as I did not want to permanently have a very high exercise level that would be difficult to maintain.

I have now achieved my target weight of 140 pounds. I think it is a little light for me. I look a little thin in the face, so I am adjusting my food intake to increase my weight a little. Because I wrote everything down, I knew the food intake level that allowed me to lose weight, to stay even or to increase weight. If I have a blowout, it does not matter as I know how much to eat to reduce any weight gained, over a week or so.

I have not recorded my intake of coffee, water or soft drinks. I did not feel the need to as my coffee is taken black without sugar, soft drinks are all diet or zero calorie and my tea consumption is around 3 cups per week which is negligible.

For the record I drink around 5 cups of coffee a day, three glasses of cola or other soft drinks and around two liters of water per day. Regarding the water, I have found that sometimes when I have felt hungry, I drank a glass of water and did not feel hungry again. Perhaps I was thirsty not hungry, or perhaps the water filled up my tummy. I don't know but it helped me.

I have been a victim of many myths over the years about losing weight. Losing weight in a hot country is easy because no one feels like eating. Losing weight in the winter is hard because hot fatty food is craved for, and a multitude of other excuses why I cannot lose weight. I want food no matter what the weather is. Hot or cold, I like food. By doing what I have done, I have as much as I like, however, I am realistic. Writing it down encourages me to be sensible. In cold months, I do eat hot foods; however, I do try to keep them to vegetable soups that are low in fat and white meats.

One thing that I believe made a massive difference to my normal failed diets is weighing everything. I have always believed that I can tell how much food I dish out by looking at it. Once I started weighing things I realized my biggest error. Two servings of equal amounts by eye, could be 30% difference by weight. With breakfast cereals, I could be 50% out. So bread, cereals, cakes, etc. I weigh.

The result is that now I control my weight. By writing everything down and weighing once a week I have learned about my body. I know how I will be affected by a night out. I also know exactly what to do to put it right. I don't see food as an enemy, I enjoy my food. I eat all sorts and have enjoyed my wine throughout. My doctor may not agree with me on the wine of course. The secret of control is knowing my tipping point and adjusting my food intake around that point. The point reduced as my weight came off me. Now I know where the tipping point is at my present weight I can adjust above or below it to control my weight quite accurately.

I do have a problem that is difficult to resolve. My weight is now great; my belly is fairly flat, not as smooth as I would like but having children does have its effect. My boobs are now smaller than I would like, and my face is somewhat thin.

I want to fatten up my face and grow back my bigger boobs, the sort that are pert and young looking and of course have a perfectly flat belly.

Why can we not choose where the fat comes from?

I don't think dieting or exercise can overcome these problems. I am happy being capable of running and walking up hills without getting out of breath and obviously being able to get clothes that fit.

As said previously I did not start out to do anything more than lose a few pounds that I had put on over Christmas. I did lose weight quite quickly and decided to write everything down, I was eating, and, to find the reason why my weight had started reducing so well. I wrote the food down a week after starting so it may not be totally accurate. It is roughly correct. From day one, it is totally accurate.

Breakfast:

- 1/2 an orange (taken from a large orange)
- 1/2 an apple
- One yogurt (or milk as some days I did not have yogurt)
- 30 to 40 grams of cereal (Preferably without sugar, However, I did start the diet with sugar-coated cereal and still lost weight)
- Two Ryvita fruit crunched crisp breads or one piece of toast.
- Two teaspoons of peanut butter, or two teaspoon of jam, or two teaspoons of golden syrup.

This breakfast was continuous during that week.

For Lunch, I either had:

- 1/2 a tin of beans with two medium slices of bread and two eggs poached,
- or one can of tuna with salad and a slice of bread,
- or soup with two slices of toast and a side salad,

- or two vegetable burgers with a side salad,
- or packet noodles with a side salad,
- or rice cakes with two eggs on and salad; they were the large rice cakes.

Now I often substituted the bread, for normal Ryvita crisp breads, because I had learned from previous diets that two Ryvita, crisp breads had the same amount of calories as one slice of bread, it also looked like I was eating more.

For the evening meal, I would have either:

- a large chicken portion with five small potatoes and vegetables,
- or a medium portion of chicken curry with a quarter of a cup of rice (that's before the rice is cooked) and side vegetables,
- or a medium portion of chili con carne with a half of a cup of rice with side vegetables, or two sausages with five small potatoes and then side vegetables.

Very often, I would stick to mostly chicken meals and have the chilies, etc. as a change.

My puddings mostly consisted of low fat jelly with a yogurt, just a jelly or a yogurt.

Then either a chocolate bar, bag of potato crisps/chips, or a bottle of wine, I chose the wine on most days.

That week of writing everything down, I lost 2lb in weight.

During the week, my observation revealed the following:

I did not eat between meals at all. I did not feel the need to.

I did not feel hungry, or that I was dieting.

I did drink squash between meals, which probably accounts for not feeling hungry.

I always ate a good breakfast to start my day.

I often substituted the bread with crisp breads, and would sometimes not eat my potatoes because I felt uncomfortable in the tummy, instead of using naan bread with curry's, I would do a side plate of vegetables instead, which gave me room to have my wine later.

Scales are imperative.

When preparing foods I would make quantities that I thought were reasonable. I knew that as I lost weight, I would need less food. How was I going to reduce my food quantities? I decided I would weigh my food, and it would then be easy to reduce quantities as my weight dropped. I was very surprised to find my quantities were nothing like I expected.

They were:

- Heavier than I thought
- Inconsistent

I could pour two servings of cereal in a dish that seemed identical to my eyes. By weight, they could be 30% different.

I realized that I must weigh everything accurately if I was going to be successful.

What follows is my daily eating diary over a six-month period with notes on how my weight was doing, how I felt, and the diet's effect on me.

The first week quantities are to be brutally honest, a guess. I started with quantities I thought seemed reasonable. I lost weight during that week so used it as a starting point for the start of my task.

My 1/2 cup of rice is 125ml and the weight of rice was 60gram.

Best of luck if you try it out.

Day 1

This diet started for me on the 9th of the 1st 2013. My weight is 175 pounds.

Breakfast:

- 1/2 an orange
- 1/2 an apple
- 30g of sugar puffs
- Two Ryvita crunch crisp breads
- Two teaspoons of jam

Lunch:

- 1/2 a tin of beans
- Four normal Ryvita crisp bread
- Two eggs poached.
- 1 low fat jelly

Evening meal:

- A large bowl of any soup
- Four Ryvita crisp breads
- 1 low fat jelly

Treats for that day:

- Half a liter of white wine.

Day 2

Breakfast:

- One peach
- 1/2 an orange
- 30g of sugar puffs
- One yogurt
- Two Ryvita crisp breads
- One teaspoon of syrup

Lunch:

- One large tin of tuna in brine (large or small.)
- A mixture of salads
- One jelly with one yogurt.

Evening meal:

- 8oz of liver (200Grams) cooked in the oven with a chopped tin of tomatoes, I added a pork stock cube with a bit of salt and pepper,
- Five small potatoes
- Loads of vegetables.

Treats:

- One bottle of white wine enjoyed throughout the evening.

Day 3

Breakfast:

- 30 grams of rice crispies
- One yogurt
- Two Ryvita crisp breads
- One level tablespoon of peanut butter
- 1/2 an orange
- 1/2 an apple

Lunch:

- A large bowl of soup
- Two slices of thick bread
- 1 low fat jelly

Evening meal:

- One large chicken portion
- 1/2 a cup of uncooked rice (1/2 cup = 125ml rice weighs 60g)
- Vegetables of choice.

Treats:

- 1/2 a bottle of 75cl wine

Notes:

The large chicken portion usually weighs about 1/2 a kilogram or 1.1lb

Day 4

Breakfast:

- 30 grams of sugar puffs
- One yogurt
- Two Ryvita crisp breads
- 2 teaspoon of syrup
- 1/2 an orange
- 1/2 an apple

Lunch:

- One piece of white fish (large)
- Mixed salad
- Four normal Ryvita crisp breads
- I added pickles (Beetroot and pickled onions)

Evening meal:

- A medium portion of chili con carne.
- 1/2 a cup of uncooked rice
- A portion of vegetables
- 1 low fat jelly

Treats:

- 1 mars bar.
- One large glass of white wine

Day 5

Breakfast:

- 30g of Sugar puffs
- One yogurt
- Two Ryvita crisp breads
- Two teaspoons of any jam
- 1/2 an apple
- 1/2 an orange

Lunch:

- A large bowl of homemade soup(vegetable)
- Two slices of thick bread
- One jelly

Evening meal:

- A large chicken portion
- 1/2 a cup of uncooked rice.
- Loads of vegetables.

Treats:

- None

Day 6

Breakfast:

- 30g of rice crispies
- 1 yogurt
- 2 Ryvita crisp breads
- 2 teaspoon of jam
- 1 peach
- 1 orange

Lunch:

- A large bowl of homemade soup
- 2 slices of thick bread
- 1 jelly

Evening meal:

- An 8oz portion of lasagne
- 1/2 a cup of uncooked rice
- A portion of vegetables

Treats:

- None

Day 7

Breakfast:

- 30g of all bran
- 1 yogurt
- 2 crisp breads
- 2 teaspoon of syrup
- 1/2 an apple
- 1/2 an orange

Lunch:

- A big bowl of soup
- 2 slices of thick bread

Evening meal:

- 1 medium sized meat pasty
- A large portion of vegetables

Treats:

- 1 brandy

Day 8

Week no 2 (Weigh day) -1.25 pound loss

Breakfast:

- 1 cereal bar (Any)
- 1 yogurt
- 2 crisp breads
- 2 teaspoons of syrup
- 1 peach

Lunch:

- Bowl of soup
- 2 slices of thick sliced bread (I am having a lot of soup for convenience really and because I am hungry, the bread is filling me up more)

Evening meal:

- 1/2 a tin of baked beans
- 2 slices of thick bread toasted
- 2 poached eggs
- 1 low fat jelly

Treats:

- 2 large glasses of white wine

Day 9

Breakfast

- 30g of sugar puffs
- 1 yogurt
- 2 crisp breads
- 2 teaspoon of syrup
- 1 peach

Lunch

- Soup again (A lot of it)
- 1 large slice of thick bread

Evening meal

- An 8oz portion of lasagne
- Loads of vegetables
- A medium bowl of ice cream

Treats

- 5 low fat biscuits
- 1 bottle of 75cl white wine

Day 10

Breakfast:

- 30g of all bran
- 1 yogurt
- 2 crisp breads
- 2 teaspoon of syrup
- 1 peach

Lunch:

- Soup again
- A large side salad

Evening meal:

- 1 vegetable burger
- 5 small potatoes
- Loads of vegetables

Treats

- 2 large glasses of wine

Day 11

Breakfast:

- 30g of all bran
- 1 yogurt
- 2 crisp breads
- 2 teaspoons of syrup
- 1/2 an apple
- 1/2 an orange

Lunch:

- 1/2 a 400g tin of beans
- 2 slices of thick bread toasted
- 2 eggs
- Side salad

Evening meal:

- 8oz portion of lasagne
- 1/4 of a cup of uncooked rice
- Unlimited vegetables

Treat:

1 brandy

Day 12

Breakfast:

- 30g sugar puffs
- 1 yogurt
- 2 crisp breads
- 1 teaspoon of jam
- 1 peach

Lunch:

- 1/2 a pack of easy cooked noodles
- 2 slices of thick bread
- side salad

Evening meal:

- 1 tin of tuna
- Side salad
- 5 small potatoes

Treats:

1 bottle of 75cl white wine enjoyed throughout the evening

Day 13

Breakfast:

- 30g of sugar puffs
- 1 yogurt
- 2 crisp breads
- 1 teaspoon of syrup
- 1/2 an apple
- 1/2 an orange

Lunch:

- 1/2 a packet of quick noodles
- 2 slices of thick bread
- Side salad

Evening Meal:

- 1 large sausage any flavor
- 5 small potatoes
- 1/2 a tin of beans
- Unlimited vegetables

Treats:

- 3 brandy measures

Day 14

Breakfast:

- 30g of sugar puffs
- 1 yogurt
- 2 crisp breads
- 1/2 a tablespoon of peanut butter
- 1 peach

Lunch:

- 8oz of lasagne
- 1 side salad

Evening meal:

- 1 vegetable burger
- 5 small potatoes
- unlimited veggies

Treat:

- 1/2 a bottle of 75cl white wine

Day 15
(weigh day) -2 pounds loss

Breakfast:

- 30 g of sugar puffs
- 1 yogurt
- 2 crisp breads
- 1 teaspoon of jam
- 1 peach

Lunch:

- Tuna and salad
- 1 jelly

Evening meal:

- 1 medium bowl of chicken curry
- 1/2 a cup of uncooked rice (125ml or 60g)
- Unlimited vegetables

Treats:

- 1/2 a bottle of 75cl white wine

Day 16

Breakfast:

- 30g of all bran
- 1 yogurt
- 2 crisp breads
- 1/2 a tablespoon of peanut butter
- 1/2 an apple
- 1/2 an orange

Lunch:

- A big bowl of homemade vegetable soup
- 2 slices of thick bread
- 1 jelly

Evening meal:

- 1 large chicken portion
- 5 small potatoes
- unlimited vegetables

Treats:

- 1 large rum and coke

Day 17

Breakfast:

- 20g of rice crispies
- 1 yogurt
- 2 crisp breads
- 1 teaspoon of jam
- 1 peach

Lunch:

- A big bowl of any soup
- 2 slices of thick bread
- Side salad

Evening meal:

- A medium portion of chilli con carne
- 1/2 a cup of uncooked rice
- unlimited vegetables

Treats:

- 1 large shortbread biscuit

Day 18

Breakfast:

- 20g of rice crispies
- 1 yogurt
- 2 rice cakes
- 1/2 a tablespoon of peanut butter
- 3 plums

Lunch:

- Homemade vegetable soup
- 2 slices of thick bread
- 1 jelly

Evening meal:

- 1 large pork chop (About 400grams)
- 5 small potatoes
- unlimited vegetables

Treats:

- 1/2 a bottle of wine
- 2 cheese flavored rice cakes (Large)

Day 19

Breakfast:

- 30g of sugar puffs
- 1 yogurt
- 1/2 a tin of mixed fruit in syrup(drain the syrup and put the mixed fruit over the cereal with the yogurt poured on the top)
- 1 rice cake
- 1/2 a teaspoon of syrup

Lunch:

- A medium portion of chicken curry
- 1/2 a cup of uncooked rice
- Unlimited vegetables

Evening meal:

- 1 big bowl of soup
- 2 thick slices of bread
- 1 jelly

Treats:

- None

Day 20

Breakfast:

- 20g of rice crispies
- 1 yogurt
- 1 large rice cake
- 1/2 a tablespoon of peanut butter
- 1 peach

Lunch:

- 1 beef stir fry(large or small it doesn't matter)
- 1 side salad

Evening meal:

- 1 medium chicken curry
- 1 portion of vegetables (no rice)

Treats:

- 1/2 a bottle of 75cl white wine

Day 21

Breakfast:

- 30g of sugar puffs
- 1 yogurt
- 1 large rice cake
- 1/2 a teaspoon of syrup
- 1 orange

Lunch:

- 1 large bowl of soup
- 2 slices of thick bread

Evening meal:

- Half a small shank of lamb (250grams of meat)
- 5 small potatoes
- unlimited vegetables

Treats:

- 2 Cadburys curly wurly chew bars

Day 22

(Weigh day) - 0.75 pounds loss, OK it doesn't seem much but its better off than on, and its comfortably coming off that's the important thing.

Breakfast:

- 30g sugar puffs
- 1 yogurt
- 2 crisp breads
- 1/2 a tablespoon of peanut butter
- 1 peach
- 1/2 an orange

Lunch:

- A medium bowl of chicken curry with rice

Evening Meal:

- 2 slices of thick bread
- 1/2 a tin of beans
- 1 egg

Treats:

- None

Day 23

Breakfast:

- 30g of sugar puffs
- 1 yogurt
- 1 large rice cake
- 1teaspoon of syrup
- 1 peach
- 1/2 an orange

Lunch:

- A big bowl of homemade soup
- 2 slices of thick bread

Evening meal:

- 1 large chicken portion
- 5 small potatoes
- unlimited vegetables

Treats:

- 1/2 a liter of white wine

Day 24

Breakfast:

- 20g of puffed wheat
- 1 yogurt
- 1/2 a tin of fruit salad (drain the juice)
- 1 peach
- 2 crisp breads
- 1 teaspoon of syrup

Lunch:

- A bowl of packet soup
- 2 slices of thick bread

Evening meal:

- One 8oz beef steak
- 5 small potatoes
- unlimited vegetables

Treats:

- 1/2 a 75cl bottle of white wine

Now I am eating a lot of soup, but it fills me up especially with the bread and I enjoy it, I Also believe it plays a great part in my weight loss too especially when I make it myself with loads of vegetables.

Day 25

Breakfast:

- Cereal and yogurt
- 1 rice cake (large)
- 1/2 a tablespoon of peanut butter
- 1 peach,

I am writing cereal and yogurt now as I know the amount of cereal and which, I will be having. I vary my cereals for interest.

Lunch:

- 1/2 a can of beans
- 2 slices of thick bread
- 2 eggs (poached)

Evening meal:

- An 8oz portion of lasagne I use both meat and vegetable lasagne
- Unlimited vegetables

Treats:

- None

Day 26

Breakfast:

- Cereal and yogurt
- 2 crisp breads
- 1/2 a tablespoon of peanut butter
- 1/2 an orange
- 1/2 an apple

Lunch:

- A bowl of soup made from a packet
- 4 rye crisp breads
- 1 jelly

Evening meal:

- 1 portion of chicken
- 5 small potatoes
- 1/2 a cup of uncooked rice

Treats:

- 1/2 a bottle of 75cl white wine

Day 27

Breakfast:

- Cereal and yogurt
- 2 crisp breads
- 1/2 a tablespoon of peanut butter
- 1/2 an apple
- 1/2 an orange

Lunch:

- 1/2 a pack of cooked noodles any flavor
- A big bowl of homemade chunky vegetable soup

Evening meal:

- 1 large piece of cod or any white fish
- Unlimited vegetables
- 1 tablespoon of mayonnaise

Treats:

- 1/2 a liter of white wine

Day 28

Breakfast:

- Cereal and yogurt
- 2 crisp breads
- 1/2 a tablespoon of peanut butter
- 1/2 a tin of mixed fruit
- 1 peach

Lunch:

- 1/2 a tin of baked beans
- 2 slices of thick bread
- 1 poached egg

Evening meal:

- 2 slices of thick bread
- 1 big dish of soup

Treats:

- None

Day 29

Weigh day -2 pounds loss

A good week last week

Breakfast:

- Cereal and yogurt
- 2 crisp breads
- 1/2 a tablespoon of peanut butter
- 1 peach

Lunch:

- A big bowl of soup made from a packet
- 2 slices of thick bread

Evening meal:

- A large piece of white fish
- 5 small potatoes
- unlimited vegetables

Treats:

- Went out in the evening and had 3 large glasses of white wine

Day 30

Breakfast:

- Cereal and yogurt
- 2 crisp breads
- 1teaspoon of jam
- 1 peach

Lunch:

- A big bowl of soup made from a packet
- 2 slices of thick bread
- 1 jelly

Evening meal:

- 1 vegetable burger
- 1/2 a cup of uncooked rice
- unlimited vegetables

Treats:

- 1/2 a liter of white wine

Day 31

Breakfast:

- Cereal and yogurt
- 2 crisp breads
- 1/2 a tablespoon of peanut butter
- 1 peach

Lunch:

- 1 small tin of tuna mashed up with-
- 1/2 a tablespoon of mayonnaise
- 4 Ryvita crisp breads
- Side salad

Evening meal:

- 1 large chicken portion
- Unlimited vegetables

Treats:

- 3 glasses of white wine

Day 32

Breakfast:

- Cereal and yogurt
- 2 Ryvita crisp breads/ or fruit crisp breads
- 2 teaspoon of honey
- 1/2 an apple
- 1/2 an orange

Lunch:

- 1 small tin of tuna mashed up with-
- 1/2 a tablespoon of mayonnaise
- 4 Ryvita crisp breads
- Side salad

Evening meal:

- 1 large pork chop
- Unlimited vegetables.

The reason I am leaving out the potatoes is because I am feeling quite bloated when I eat them at the moment,

Treats:

- 1/2 a liter of white wine

You may think I am having a lot of wine, but I am spreading it out through the evening and at this stage I prefer it rather than chocolate bars. I try not to have both; I either have one or the other.

Day 33

Breakfast:

- Cereal and yogurt
- 2 Ryvita crisp breads
- 1/2 a tablespoon of peanut butter
- 1 apple
- 1/2 an orange

Lunch:

- 1 bowl of soup made from a packet
- 4 Ryvita crisp breads
- Side salad

Evening Meal:

- 4 Ryvita crisp breads
- 1/2 a tin of baked beans
- 2 eggs poached

Treats:

- 1/2 a liter of white wine enjoyed throughout the evening

Day 34

Breakfast:

- Cereal and yogurt
- 2 Ryvita crisp breads
- 1/2 a tablespoon of peanut butter
- 1/2 an apple
- 1/2 an orange

Lunch:

- A bowl of soup made from a packet
- 2 Ryvita crisp breads
- 1 large rice cake

Evening meal:

- 1 large chicken portion
- 5 small potatoes
- Unlimited vegetables

Treats:

- 1/2 a liter of white wine enjoyed throughout the evening

Day 35

Breakfast:

- Cereal and yogurt
- 2 crisp breads
- 2 teaspoon of honey
- 1/2 an apple
- 1/2 an orange

Lunch:

- 1 big bowl of soup
- 4 Ryvita crisp breads
- Side salad

Evening meal:

- 1 large tin of tuna
- 5 small potatoes
- side salad
- 1/2 a tablespoon of mayonnaise

Treats:

- 1/2 a liter of white wine enjoyed throughout the evening

Day 36

Weigh Day -1 pound loss

Wow another pound off comfortably, that's 6 and a half pounds in total so far. I have decided to keep writing it down just in case I do not lose any one week and I can look back on what I have eaten that week and decide what to cut out if I need too.
Breakfast:

- Cereal and yogurt
- 2 crisp breads
- 1/2 a tablespoon of peanut butter
- 1/2 an apple
- 1/2 an orange

Lunch:

- Tuna and salad
- 1 jelly

Evening meal:

- 1 vegetable burger
- 5 small potatoes
- unlimited vegetables
- 3 plums
-
Treats:

- 1/2 a liter of white wine enjoyed throughout the evening

Day 37

Breakfast:

- Cereal and yogurt
- 2 Ryvita crisp breads
- 1/2 a tablespoon of peanut butter
- 1 peach

Lunch:

- 2 slices of thick bread
- 2 poached eggs

Evening meal:

- 1 chicken portion
- 1/2 a cup of uncooked rice
- Unlimited vegetables

Treats:

- 2 large glasses of white wine

Day 38

Breakfast:

- Cereal and yogurt
- 2 Ryvita crisp breads
- 2 teaspoon of honey
- 1 peach

Lunch:

- 1 big bowl of soup made from a packet
- 4 crisp breads

Evening meal:

- A medium plateful of home made chilli con carne
- Unlimited vegetables

Treats:

- 1/2 a liter of white wine enjoyed throughout the evening

Day 39

Breakfast:

- Cereal and yogurt
- 1 large rice cake
- 1 teaspoon of honey
- 1 peach
- 1/2 an orange

Lunch:

- 4 Ryvita crisp breads
- 2 eggs

Evening meal:

- 1 large tin of tuna
- 5 small potatoes
- Unlimited vegetables
- 3 plums

Treats:

- 1/2 a liter of white wine

Day 40

Breakfast:

- Cereal and yogurt
- 2 crisp breads
- 2 teaspoon of honey
- 1 orange
- 1/2 an apple

Lunch:

- 1 large bowl of soup made from a packet (any flavor)
- 4 Ryvita crisp breads

Evening meal:

- 1 large chicken portion
- 5 small potatoes
- unlimited vegetables

Treats:

- 1 large glass of wine

Day 41

Breakfast:

- Cereal and yogurt
- 2 Ryvita crisp breads
- 1 teaspoon of jam
- 1 peach

Lunch:

- 4 Ryvita crisp breads
- 2 eggs

Evening meal:

- A portion of homemade chilli con carne
- 1/2 a cup of uncooked rice
- Unlimited vegetables

Treats:

- None

Day 42

Breakfast:

- Cereal and yogurt
- 2 Ryvita crisp breads
- 1 teaspoon of honey
- 1 apple
- 1/2 an orange

Lunch:

- 1 vegetable burger
- A side salad
- 4 crisp breads

Evening meal:

- 1 large chicken portion
- 5 small potatoes
- Unlimited vegetables

Treats:

- None

Day 43

Weigh day -4 pounds lost

Another fantastic weight loss! I will continue as I am at present.

Breakfast:

- Cereal and yogurt
- 2 Ryvita crisp breads
- 1/2 a tin of fruit with juice drained
- 1 teaspoon of jam

Lunch:

- 2 Ryvita crisp breads
- 1 poached egg
- A side salad

Evening meal:

- 8oz of liver cooked in the oven with a tin of tomatoes 1 beef stock cube mixed in with a little salt and pepper.
- 5 small potatoes
- Unlimited vegetables

Treats:

- 1/2 a liter of white wine enjoyed throughout the evening

Day 44

Breakfast:

- Cereal and yogurt
- 2 Ryvita crisp breads
- 1 teaspoon of honey
- 1 peach

Lunch:

- 1 bowl of soup made up from a packet
- 4 Ryvita crisp breads
- 1 jelly

Evening meal:

- Tuna and salad
- 5 small potatoes

Treats:

- 1/2 a liter of white wine

Day 45

Breakfast:

- Cereal and yogurt
- 1 large rice cake
- Tsp of jam
- 1 peach

Lunch:

- 1 vegetable burger
- 2 crisp breads
- 1 bowl of soup

Evening meal:

- 1 chicken portion
- 1/2 a cup of uncooked rice
- unlimited veg

Treats:

- 1 bottle of 75cl white wine enjoyed throughout the evening

Day 46

I have decided to start going to the gym at this stage to give me a boost

Breakfast:

- Cereal and yogurt
- 2 Ryvita crisp breads
- 1 teaspoon of honey
- 1 peach

Lunch:

- 1 vegetable burger with salad
- 1 jelly

Evening meal:

- A piece of white fish cooked without fat
- 5 small potatoes
- unlimited vegetables
- 2 Ryvita crisp breads

Treats:

- 1/2 a bottle of 75cl wine

Day 47

Ouch I feel heavy today after being at the gym and a little sore we will see.

Breakfast:

- Cereal and yogurt
- 2 Ryvita crisp breads
- 2 teaspoon of jam
- 1 peach

Lunch:

- 1 piece of fish (white)
- A side salad
- 2 Ryvita crisp breads

Evening meal:

- 1 chicken portion
- unlimited veg
- 1/2 a cup of uncooked rice

Treats:

- None

Day 48

Well someone said to me today expect your weight loss to slow down now you have started at the gym, when I asked why they said its because your fat will disintegrate and you will gain more muscle until your body settles down, ha I said my weight loss is slow anyway so it shouldn't make much difference (we will see)

Breakfast:

- Cereal and yogurt
- 2 Ryvita crisp breads
- 2 teaspoon of jam
- 1 peach

Lunch:

- 1 large bowl of soup
- 4 Ryvita crisp breads
- 1 jelly

Evening meal:

- 1/2 a tin of beans
- 2 eggs
- 4 Ryvita crisp breads.

Treats:

- 1/2 a liter of white wine

Now what I do with this meal is place all four crisp breads on a dinner plate, then I pour the baked beans over them, then I put the two poached eggs on the top of them. Sometimes I am able to pick the crisp breads up and eat them with some beans on top, or I just use a knife and fork to cut them as if you are just eating toast,(lovely) and you feel like you are eating more.

Day 49

Going to have my breakfast then I will wait 2 hours then go to the gym.

Breakfast:

- Cereal and yogurt
- 2 Ryvita fruit crisp breads
- 1 teaspoon of syrup
- 1 peach

Lunch:

- A large bowl of homemade vegetable soup
- 2 slices of thick bread (I am hungry Its the gym I reckon)
- 1 jelly and yogurt

Evening meal:

- 1 Large chicken portion
- 5 small potatoes
- Unlimited vegetables

Treats:

- 1/2 a 75cl bottle of white wine

Day 50

Weigh day +1 pound

Hey hey hey, what's going on here I ask! ummm must be my body adapting to the gym I will not give up.

Breakfast:

- Cereal and yogurt
- 2 Ryvita fruit crisp breads
- 1 teaspoon of jam
- 1 orange

Lunch:

- A large bowl of homemade vegetable soup
- 4 Ryvita crisp breads
- 1 jelly

Evening meal:

- Medium bowl of bolognaise with a medium bowl of pasta.
- Unlimited vegetables

Treats:

- 1 bottle of 75cl white wine enjoyed throughout the evening

Day 51

Gym day again today I have decided to go every two days, it did hurt at first but not now, Cardiovascular is good for keeping up with the weight loss. Followed by a few strengthening exercises.

Breakfast:

- Cereal and yogurt
- 2 normal Ryvita crisp breads
- 1 teaspoon of syrup
- 1/2 an apple
- 1/2 an orange

Lunch:

- 2 poached eggs
- 1/2 a tin of beans
- 4 Ryvita crisp breads

Evening meal:

- 1 large chicken portion
- 5 small potatoes
- Unlimited vegetables
- 1 peach

Treats:

- 2 glasses of white wine

Day 52

Breakfast:

- Cereal and yogurt
- 1 large Rice cake
- 1 teaspoon of syrup
- 1/2 a tin of mixed fruit (juice drained)

Lunch:

- A medium piece of white fish cooked without fat
- A large portion of salad

Evening meal:

- 1 vegetable burger
- 1/2 a cup of uncooked rice
- Unlimited vegetables

Treats:

- 1/2 a bottle of 75cl white wine

Day 53

Gym Day

Breakfast:

- Cereal and yogurt
- 2 Ryvita crisp breads
- 1 teaspoon of jam
- 1/2 a tin of mixed fruit (Juice drained)

Lunch:

- A big bowl of packet made soup
- 4 Ryvita crisp breads
- 1 jelly

Evening meal:

- 1 large portion of chicken
- 5 Small potatoes
- Unlimited vegetables

Treats:

- 1/2 a bottle of 75cl white wine

Day 54

Breakfast:

- Cereal and yogurt
- 1 peach
- 1/2 an orange
- 1 Ryvita fruit crisp bread
- 1 teaspoon of syrup

Lunch:

- 1/2 a tin of beans
- 2 eggs
- 4 Ryvita crisp breads

Evening meal:

- Medium portion of white fish
- Unlimited vegetables

Treats:

- 2 large glasses of white wine

Day 55

Breakfast:

- Cereal and yogurt
- 2 Ryvita crisp breads
- 1 teaspoon of syrup
- 1/2 a tin of mixed fruit (juice drained)

Lunch:

- A medium portion of any flavor pizza
- 1 large bowl of soup
- 1 jelly

Evening meal:

- 1 medium pork chop (200 grams)
- Lots of salad

Treats:

- 1 bottle of 75cl white wine enjoyed throughout the evening

Day 56

Breakfast:

- Cereal and yogurt
- 1 large rice cake
- 1 teaspoon of syrup
- 1/2 a tin of mixed fruit (Juice drained)

Lunch:

- 4 Ryvita crisp breads
- 2 poached eggs

Evening meal:

- 1 chicken portion
- Unlimited salad

Treats:

- 1/2 a liter of white wine

Day 57

Weigh day - 2 pounds loss

That's more like it, my body must have settled down as I am going to the gym regularly now.

Breakfast:

- Cereal and yogurt
- 1 large rice cake
- 1 Ryvita crisp bread
- 1 teaspoon of syrup (It doesn't matter if I go over with the syrup as long as I have enough to spread on each crisp bread evenly) I am using as a guide 1 teaspoon
- 1/2 a tin of mixed fruit (juice drained)

Lunch:

- 2 large rice cakes
- 1 bowl of packet made soup

Evening meal:

- 1 medium bowl of chicken curry
- 1/2 a cup of uncooked rice
- Unlimited vegetables

Treats:

- 1/2 a liter of white wine

Day 58

Breakfast:

- cereal and yogurt
- 1 large rice cake
- 1 teaspoon of jam
- 1/2 an apple
- 1/2 an orange
- 1 plum

Lunch:

- A bowl of packet made soup
- 2 slices of thick bread
- 1 jelly

Evening meal:

- 1 large chicken portion
- 5 small potatoes
- Unlimited vegetables

Treats:

- 1/2 a bottle of 75cl white wine
- 1 apple

Day 59

Breakfast:

- Cereal and yogurt
- 1 large Rice cake
- 1 teaspoon of syrup
- 1 peach
- 1/2 an orange

Lunch:

- 2 slices of thick bread toasted
- 2 poached eggs
- 1 jelly

Evening meal:

- 1 chicken portion
- 5 small potatoes
- Unlimited vegetables

Treats:

- 1/2 a bottle of 75cl white wine

Day 60

Breakfast:

- Cereal and yogurt
- 1 large Rice cake
- 1 teaspoon of jam
- 1 peach

Lunch:

- 1 packet of noodles cooked

Evening meal:

- 1 large chicken portion
- Unlimited vegetables

Treats:

- 1 bottle of 75cl white wine enjoyed throughout the evening
- 1/2 a pint glass of cider

Day 61

Breakfast:

- Cereal and yogurt
- 1 Rice cake
- 1 teaspoon of syrup
- 1 peach

Lunch:

- A large bowl of packet made soup
- 2 slices of thick bread
- 1 jelly

Evening meal:

- A medium bowl of spaghetti Carbonara
- Side salad

Treats:

- 1 glass of cider
- 1/2 a bottle of 75cl wine

Day 62

Breakfast:

- Cereal and yogurt
- 2 crisp breads
- 1 teaspoon of jam
- 1 peach

Lunch:

- Medium bowl of pasta
- side salad
- Jelly

Evening meal:

- 1 large chicken portion
- 5 small potatoes
- unlimited vegetables

Treats:

- 1/2 a bottle of 75cl white wine

Day 63

Breakfast:

- Cereal and yogurt
- 2 crisp breads
- 1 teaspoon of syrup
- 1 peach

Lunch:

- 1 packet of noodles cooked
- 2 crisp breads

Evening meal:

- 1 large chicken portion
- vegetables
- 1/2 a cup of uncooked rice

Treats:

- 1/2 a bottle of 75cl white wine

Day 64

Weigh day -1.25 pounds Loss

Breakfast:

- Cereal and yogurt
- 1 peach
- 2 crisp breads
- 1 teaspoon of jam

Lunch:

- 1 large bowl of soup
- 4 Ryvita crisp breads

Evening meal:

- 1 large chicken portion
- 5 small potatoes
- Unlimited vegetables

Treats:

- None

Day 65

Breakfast:

- Cereal and yogurt
- 1 large rice cake
- 1 teaspoon of syrup
- 1 peach

Lunch:

- 1 large bowl of soup
- 4 Ryvita crisp breads

Evening meal:

- Medium chicken portion
- Vegetables
- 5 small potatoes

Treats:

- 1/2 a bottle of 75cl white wine
- 1 mars bar

Day 66

Breakfast:

- Cereal and yogurt
- 1 large rice cake
- 1 teaspoon of syrup
- 1 peach
- 1/2 an orange

Lunch:

- 1/2 a tin of baked beans
- 2 poached eggs
- 4 Ryvita crisp breads

Evening meal:

- 1 vegetable burger
- vegetables
- 1/2 a cup of uncooked rice

Treats:

- 1/2 a bottle of 75cl white wine

Day 67

Breakfast:

- Cereal and yogurt
- 2 crisp breads
- 1 teaspoon of syrup
- 1 peach

Lunch:

- 1 large bowl of soup
- 4 Ryvita crisp breads

Evening meal:

- 1 medium piece of fish(200grams)
- 5 small potatoes
- unlimited vegetables

Treats:

- 1 bottle of 75cl white wine

Day 68

Breakfast:

- Cereal and yogurt
- 2 crisp breads
- 1 teaspoon of jam
- 1 peach

Lunch:

- A big bowl of any soup
- 1 thick piece of bread

Evening meal:

- 1 medium bowl of chili con carne
- 1 cup of uncooked rice

Treats:

- 4 squares of milk chocolate
- 1 small beer

Day 69

Breakfast:

- Cereal and yogurt
- 1 orange
- 2 crisp breads
- 1 teaspoon of syrup

Lunch:

- Tuna and salad
- Small piece of pizza any sort

Evening meal:

- 1 small chicken leg(200g)
- 1 vegetable burger
- unlimited vegetables

Treats:

- 1 bottle of 75cl wine enjoyed throughout the evening

Day 70

Breakfast:

- Cereal and yogurt
- 1 piece of fruit (Any)
- 2 crisp breads
- 1 teaspoon of jam

Lunch:

- 1 medium piece of white fish
- Loads of salad

Evening meal:

- 1 vegetable burger
- 5 small potatoes
- unlimited vegetables
- 1 Tablespoon of onion relish

Treats:

- 1 bottle of 75cl wine
- 4 squares of milk chocolate

Day 71

Weigh day-1 and a 1/4 pound

Breakfast

- Cereal and yogurt
- 1/2 an apple
- 1/2 an orange
- 2 crisp breads
- 1 teaspoon of syrup

Lunch
- Tuna and salad

Evening meal

- 1 medium bowl of chilli
- 1 cupful of uncooked rice
- Unlimited vegetables

Treats
- 1/2 a bottle of 75cl white wine

Day 72

Breakfast:

- Cereal and yogurt
- 1 rice cake
- 1 teaspoon of jam
- 1 piece of fruit

Lunch:

- 1/2 a tin of baked beans
- 2 poached eggs
- 4 Ryvita crisp breads

Evening Meal:

- 1 big bowl of soup
- 4 crisp breads

Treats:

- 1 bottle of 75cl white wine enjoyed throughout the evening

Day 73

Breakfast:

- Cereal and yogurt
- 2 crisp breads
- 1 teaspoon of syrup
- 1 orange

Lunch:

- 1 big bowl of any soup
- 4 Ryvita crisp breads
- 1 dish of low fat jelly

Evening meal:

- 1 piece of medium white fish
- unlimited vegetables

Treats:

- 1 bottle of 75cl white wine
- 1 mars bar

Day 74

Breakfast:

- Cereal and yogurt
- 1 peach
- 1 small orange
- 2 crisp breads
- 1 teaspoon of jam

Lunch:

- 1 big bowl of any soup
- 4 crisp breads

Evening meal:

- Tuna and salad

Treats:

- 1 bottle of 75cl white wine

Day 75

Breakfast:

- Cereal and yogurt
- 1 peach
- 2 crisp breads
- 1 teaspoon of syrup

Lunch

- 1 big bowl of soup
- 4 crisp breads

Evening meal

- Chilli con carne and rice

Treats:

- 1 mars bar
- 1/2 a bottle of 75cl white wine

Day 76

Breakfast:

- Cereal and yogurt
- 2 crisp breads
- 1 teaspoon of syrup
- 1 piece of fruit

Lunch:

- 1 big bowl of any soup
- 4 crisp breads

Evening meal:

- Tuna and salad

Treats:

- 1/2 a bottle of 75cl white wine

Day 77

Breakfast:

- Cereal and yogurt
- 2 crisp breads
- 1teaspoon of syrup
- 1 piece of any fruit

Lunch:

- 1/2 a pack of flavored noodles cooked
- 4 crisp breads

Evening meal:

- 1 medium piece of white fish
- 5 small potatoes
- Unlimited vegetables

Treats:

- 1/2 a bottle of 75cl white wine

Day 78

Weigh day -1.5 a pound

Breakfast:

- Cereal and yogurt
- 2 crisp breads
- 1 piece of any fruit
- 1 teaspoon of syrup

Lunch:

- 1 piece of white fish
- 4 crisp breads

Evening meal:

- 2 pork sausages
- 5 small potatoes
- Unlimited vegetables

Treats:

- None

Day 79

Breakfast:

- Cereal and yogurt
- 1 piece of fruit
- 2 Ryvita fruit crisp breads
- 1 teaspoon of syrup

Lunch:

- Tuna and salad

Evening meal:

- 1 vegetable burger
- 5 small potatoes
- Unlimited vegetables

Treats:

- 1 bottle of 75cl white wine enjoyed throughout the evening

Day 80

Breakfast:

- Cereal and yogurt
- 1 orange
- 1 apple
- 2 crisp breads
- 1 teaspoon of syrup

Lunch:

- 1 large bowl of any soup
- 4 crisp breads

Evening meal:

- Chilli con carne
- 1 cup of uncooked rice
- Unlimited vegetables

Treats:

- 1 mars bar

Day 81

Breakfast:

- Cereal and yogurt
- 2 Ryvita fruit crisp breads
- 1 teaspoon of syrup
- 1 peach
- 1 small orange

Lunch:

- 1 piece of white fish
- 4 crisp breads

Evening meal:

- 1 large sausage
- 5 small potatoes
- Unlimited vegetables

Treats:

- 1/2 a bottle of 75cl white wine

Day 82

Breakfast:

- Cereal and yogurt
- 2 Ryvita fruit crisp breads
- 1 teaspoon of syrup
- 1 piece of fruit

Lunch:

- Tuna and salad

Evening meal:

- 1/2 a pack of flavored noodles
- Unlimited vegetables
- 4 crisp breads

Treats:

- None

Day 83

Breakfast:

- Cereal and yogurt
- 1 large rice cake
- 1 teaspoon of syrup
- 1 peach
- 1 small orange

Lunch:

- 4 crisp breads
- 1/2 a tin of baked beans
- 2 poached eggs

Evening meal:

- Chilli con carne
- 1 cup of uncooked rice
- Unlimited vegetables

Treats:

- None

Day 84

Breakfast:

- Cereal and yogurt
- 1 large rice cake
- 1 teaspoon of syrup
- 1 peach
- 1 small orange

Lunch:

- Large bowl of any soup
- 4 crisp breads
- A dish of low fat jelly

Evening meal:

- 1 large chicken portion
- 5 small potatoes
- Unlimited vegetables

Treats:

- 1/2 a bottle of 75cl white wine

Day 85

Weigh day-0.75 pound

Breakfast:

- Cereal and yogurt
- 2 Ryvita fruit crisp breads
- 1 teaspoon of syrup
- 1 apple
- 1 small orange

Lunch:

- Tuna and salad

Evening meal:

- 1 large chicken portion
- 5 small potatoes
- Unlimited vegetables

Treats:

- 1/2 a bottle of 75cl white wine

Day 86

Breakfast:

- Cereal and yogurt
- 2 Ryvita fruit crisp breads
- 1 teaspoon of syrup
- 1 pear
- 1 small orange

Lunch:

- 1 bowl of soup
- 1 slice of thick bread
- 1 mars bar

Evening meal:

- 1 chicken portion
- 5 small potatoes
- Unlimited vegetables

Treats:

- None

Day 87

Breakfast:

- Cereal and yogurt
- 1 slice of thick bread
- 1 teaspoon of jam
- 1 apple
- 1 small orange

Lunch:

- 2 slices of medium bread
- 1/2 a tin of baked beans
- A dish of low fat jelly

Evening meal:

- 1 vegetable burger
- 5 small potatoes
- Unlimited vegetables
- 1/2 a tablespoon of mayonnaise

Treats:

- None

Day 88

Breakfast:

- Cereal and yogurt
- 2 Ryvita fruit crisp breads
- 1 teaspoon of jam

Lunch:

- 1 bowl of soup
- 4 crisp breads

Evening meal:

- 1 piece of white fish
- 5 small potatoes
- Unlimited vegetables

Treats:

- 1/2 a bottle of 75cl white wine

Day 89

Breakfast:

- Cereal and yogurt
- 2 Ryvita fruit crisp breads
- 1 teaspoon of jam
- 1 peach
- 1 small orange

Lunch:

- 1 medium sized baked potato
- 1 tin of tuna(medium) mixed with
- 1 tablespoon of mayonnaise

Evening meal:

- 1 chicken portion
- Unlimited vegetables

Treats:

- 1/2 a bottle of 75cl white wine

Day 90

Breakfast:

- Cereal and yogurt
- 2 Ryvita fruit crisp breads
- 1 teaspoon of jam
- 1 peach
- 1 small orange

Lunch:

- Tuna salad

Evening meal:

- 1 medium chicken portion
- 5 small potatoes
- Unlimited vegetables

Treats:

- 1 bottle of 75cl white wine

Day 91

Breakfast:

- Cereal and yogurt
- 2 Ryvita fruit crisp breads
- 1 teaspoon of jam
- 1 peach

Lunch:

- 1 medium baked potato mixed with
- 1 tin of tuna and
- 1 tablespoon of mayonnaise

Evening meal:

- 2 slices of thick bread toasted
- 2 cheese triangles spread on the toast
- 2 poached eggs

Treats:

- None

Day 92

Weigh day-1.75 pounds loss

Breakfast:

- Cereal and yogurt
- 2 slices of thick bread
- 1 teaspoon of jam
- 1 orange

Lunch:

- 1 bowl of soup
- 4 crisp breads

Evening meal:

- 5 oz. of steak
- 1 egg
- 3 small potatoes
- Unlimited vegetables

Treats:

- None

Day 93

Breakfast:

- Cereal and yogurt
- 1 slice of thick bread
- 1 teaspoon of jam
- 1 peach

Lunch:

- 1 pack of flavored noodles cooked
- A bowl of salad

Evening meal:

- 2 slices of thick bread
- 1/2 a tin of baked beans
- A dish of low fat jelly

Treats:

- None

Day 94

Breakfast:

- Cereal and yogurt
- 1 slice of toast
- 1 teaspoon of jam
- 1 peach

Lunch:

- 2 medium slices of bread toasted
- 1/2 a tin of beans
- 1 egg poached

Evening meal:

- 1 medium sausage
- 4 small potatoes
- Unlimited salad

Treats:

- 1/2 a bottle of 75cl white wine

Day 95

Breakfast:

- Cereal and yogurt
- 1 slice of toast
- 1 teaspoon of jam
- 1 large orange

Lunch:

- 2 slices of thick bread toasted
- 2 poached eggs

Evening meal:

- 1 large chicken portion
- 1 cup of uncooked rice
- Unlimited vegetables
- 1 tablespoon of mayonnaise

Treats:

- 1 large glass of white wine

Day 96

Breakfast:

- Cereal and yogurt
- 1 slice of thick bread toasted
- 1 teaspoon of jam
- 1 piece of any fruit

Lunch:

- 2 slices of thick bread toasted
- 2 poached eggs

Evening meal:

- 1 large pork chop
- 1 cupful of uncooked rice
- Unlimited vegetables

Treats:

- 1 Apple

Day 97

Breakfast:

- Cereal and yogurt
- 1/2 a tin of tinned fruit drained
- 1 orange
- 2 crisp breads
- 1 teaspoon of syrup

Lunch:

- Tuna and salad

Evening meal:

- 1 beef burger
- 5 small potatoes
- Unlimited vegetables

Treats:

- 2 glasses of wine

Day 98

Breakfast:

- Cereal and yogurt
- 2 crisp breads
- 1 teaspoon of syrup
- 1 piece of fruit

Lunch:

- Tuna and salad
- 2 rice cakes

Evening meal:

- 1 chicken portion
- 1 cupful of uncooked rice
- Unlimited vegetables

Treats:

- None

Day 99

Weigh day-1.75 pounds loss

The weight is coming off slowly but surely at a steady pace.

Breakfast:

- Cereal and yogurt
- 2 crisp breads
- 1 teaspoon of syrup
- 1 piece of fruit

Lunch:

- 1 large piece of white fish
- Lots of salad

Evening meal:

- Large chicken portion
- 5 small potatoes
- Unlimited vegetables
- 1 orange

Treats:

- 1 large white wine

Day 100

Breakfast:

- Cereal and yogurt
- 1 large rice cake
- 1 teaspoon of jam
- 1 peach
- 1 small orange

Lunch:

- Tuna and salad
- 1 slice of bread

Evening meal:

- 1 vegetable burger
- Unlimited vegetables

Treats:

- 2 large glasses of red wine

Day 101

Breakfast:

- Cereal and yogurt
- 2 Ryvita fruit crisp breads
- 1 teaspoon of syrup
- 1 piece of fruit

Lunch:

- 1 Large chicken portion
- 1 cup of uncooked rice
- Unlimited vegetables

At this stage I have swopped my meals around because of going to the gym in the evening.

Evening meal:

- 1 large bowl of soup
- 2 slices of thick bread

Treats:

- 1 large glass of wine
- 1 gin and tonic

Day 102

Breakfast:

- Cereal and yogurt
- 2 fruit Ryvita crisp bread
- 1 teaspoon of syrup
- 1 peach
- 1 small orange

Lunch:

- 1 large bowl of soup
- 2 thick slices of bread

Evening meal:

- 1 large chicken portion
- 5 small potatoes
- Unlimited vegetables

Treats:
- 1/2 a bottle of 75cl white wine

Day 103

Breakfast:

- Cereal and yogurt
- 2 Ryvita fruit crisp breads
- 2 teaspoon of jam
- 1 small banana
- 1 small orange

Lunch:

- Large tin of tuna
- Salad

Evening meal:

- 2 large rice cakes
- 2 poached eggs
- 1/2 a tin of baked beans

Treats:

- 1 bottle of 75cl white wine

Day 104

Breakfast:

- Cereal and yogurt
- 2 Ryvita fruit crisp breads
- 1 tablespoon of peanut butter
- 1 apple
- 1 orange

Lunch:

- Tuna and salad

Evening meal:

- Medium portion of chicken curry with rice
- Unlimited vegetables

Treats:

- None

Day 105

Breakfast:

- Cereal and yogurt
- 2 large rice cakes
- 2 teaspoon of syrup
- 1 peach
- 1 orange

Lunch:

- 2 large rice cakes
- 2 slices of ham
- Lots of salad

Evening meal:

- 1 chicken portion
- Unlimited vegetables

Treats:

- 1/2 a bottle of 75cl white wine

Day 106

Weigh day-1.5 pounds

Breakfast:

- Cereal and yogurt
- 2 Ryvita fruit crisp breads
- 1 teaspoon of syrup
- 1 piece of any fruit

Lunch:

- 4 crisp breads
- 1/2 a tin of beans
- 2 poached eggs

Evening meal:

- Medium bowl of any meat curry
- 1/2 cup of uncooked rice
- Unlimited vegetables

Treats:

- None

Day 107

Breakfast:

- Cereal and yogurt
- 2 Ryvita fruit crisp breads
- 1 teaspoon of syrup
- 1/2 a tin of mixed fruit juice drained
- 1 peach

Lunch:

- 4 crisp breads
- 1 large bowl of soup

Evening meal:

- 1 medium bowl of chilli
- 1/2 cup of uncooked rice

Treats:

- None

Day 108

Breakfast:

- Cereal and yogurt
- 1 peach
- Small Glass of orange juice
- 2 normal crisp breads
- 1/2 a tablespoon of peanut butter

Lunch:

- 2 Medium slices of liver cooked however you want it
- 1/2 cup of uncooked rice
- Unlimited vegetables

Evening meal:

- Large bowl of soup
- 2 slices of thick bread

Treats:

- 1/2 a liter of white wine
- 2 small whiskeys

Day 109

Breakfast:

- Cereal and yogurt
- 2 normal crisp breads
- 1/2 a tablespoon of peanut butter
- 1 peach

Lunch:

- 2 slices of thick bread
- 1/2 a tin of baked beans
- 2 poached eggs

Evening Meal:

- Large bowl of soup
- 2 thick slices of bread

Treats:

- 1/2 a liter of white wine
- 2 medium wines
- 1 whiskey

Day 110

Breakfast:

- Cereal and yogurt
- 2 crisp breads
- 1 teaspoon of syrup, 2 pieces of fruit (Any)

Lunch:

- A big bowl of soup
- 2 slices of thick bread

Evening meal:

- 1 large chicken portion
- 1/2 cup of uncooked rice
- Unlimited vegetables

Treats:

- 1/2 a liter of white wine

Day 111

Breakfast:

- Cereal and yogurt
- 2 Ryvita fruit crisp breads
- 1 teaspoon of syrup
- 1 peach
- 1 small orange

The teaspoon of syrup is just a guide. A little more did not matter as it is hard to measure.

Lunch:

- 1 large piece of white fish
- Unlimited salad

Evening meal:

- 1 medium chicken portion
- 5 small potatoes
- Unlimited vegetables
- 1 peach

Treats:

- None

Day 112

Breakfast:

- Cereal and yogurt
- 1 crisp bread
- 1 teaspoon of syrup
- 1/2 a tin of mixed fruit juice drained

Lunch:

- 1 vegetable burger
- Unlimited salad

Evening meal:

- 1 medium chicken portion
- Unlimited vegetables

Treats:

- 1 bottle of 75cl white wine
- 1 dish of homemade ice cream

Day 113

Weigh day-1.5 pounds

Breakfast:

- Cereal and yogurt
- 2 normal crisp breads
- 1 teaspoon of syrup
- 1 peach
- 1 small orange

Lunch:

- 1 large bowl of soup
- 2 thick slices of bread

Evening meal:

- 1 large chicken portion
- 5 small potatoes
- Unlimited vegetables

Treats:

- 1/2 a bottle of 75cl white wine
- 1 mars bar

Day 114

Breakfast:

- Cereal and yogurt
- 1 Ryvita fruit crisp bread
- 1 teaspoon of syrup
- 2 pieces of fruit

Lunch:

- Tuna and salad

Evening meal:

- 1 vegetable burger
- 1/2 cup of uncooked rice
- Unlimited vegetables

Treats:

- 1 bottle of 75cl white wine

Day 115

Breakfast:

- Cereal and yogurt
- 2 normal crisp breads
- 1/2 a tablespoon of peanut butter
- 1 peach
- 1 small orange

Lunch:

- 4 crisp breads
- 2 poached eggs

Evening meal:

- 1 large chicken portion
- Unlimited vegetables

Treats:

- 1/2 a bottle of 75cl white wine

Day 116

Breakfast:

- Cereal and yogurt
- 2 Ryvita crisp breads
- 1 teaspoon of syrup
- 1 peach
- 1 small orange

Lunch:

- 1/2 a tin of baked beans
- 4 Ryvita crisp breads

Evening meal:

- 1 medium bowl of chilli
- Unlimited vegetables
- No rice

Treats:

- 1/2 a bottle of 75cl white wine

Day 117

Breakfast:

- Cereal and yogurt
- 2 Ryvita fruit crisp breads
- 1 teaspoon of syrup
- 1 peach
- 1 small orange

Lunch;

- Small tin of tuna with salad and
- 1 tablespoon of mayonnaise

Evening meal:

- 1 Medium bowl of curry
- No rice
- Unlimited vegetables
- 4 crisp breads

Treats:

- 1 mars bar

Day 118

Breakfast:

- Cereal and yogurt
- 2 Ryvita fruit crisp breads
- 1 teaspoon of syrup
- 1 peach
- 1 small orange

Lunch:

- 4 crisp breads
- 1/2 a tin of baked beans

Evening meal:

- 1 large sausage
- 1/2 cup of uncooked rice
- Unlimited vegetables

Treats:

- 1/2 a bottle of 75cl white wine

Day 119

Breakfast:

- Cereal and yogurt
- 2 Ryvita fruit crisp breads
- 1 teaspoon of syrup
- 1 peach
- 1 small orange

Lunch:

- Tuna and salad
- 4 crisp breads

Evening meal:

- 1 small chicken portion
- 5 small potatoes
- Unlimited vegetables

Treats:

- 1 bottle of 75cl white wine

Day 120

Weigh day +0.25 pound gain OOPS!

I had better be careful; however it is only 1/4 of a pound

Breakfast:

- Cereal and yogurt
- 1 large rice cake
- 1/2 a tablespoon of peanut butter
- 1 peach
- 1 small orange

Lunch:

- 1 large bowl of soup
- 2 thick slices of bread

Evening meal:

- 1 large chicken portion
- 5 small potatoes
- Unlimited vegetables

Treats:

- None

Day 121

Breakfast:

- Cereal and yogurt
- 1 peach
- 2 normal crisp breads
- 1/2 a tablespoon of peanut butter

Lunch:

- 1/2 a tin of baked beans
- 2 slices of thick bread
- 2 poached eggs

Evening meal:

- 1 large bowl of soup
- 2 thick slices of bread

Treats:

- 1/2 a 75cl bottle of white wine

Day 122

Breakfast:

- Cereal and yogurt
- 1 peach
- 2 normal crisp breads
- 1 teaspoon of syrup

Lunch:

- Tuna and salad

Evening meal:

- 2 medium slices of liver cooked to how you want it
- 5 small potatoes
- Unlimited vegetables

Treats:

- 1 bottle of 75cl white wine

Day 123

Breakfast:

- Cereal and yogurt
- 2 normal crisp breads
- 1/2 a tablespoon of peanut butter
- 1 peach

Lunch:

- 1 large bowl of soup
- 2 slices of thick bread
- 2 large glasses of wine

Evening meal:

- 1 medium piece of chicken
- A portion of homemade moussaka (Greek dish)
- 1/2 cup of uncooked rice

Treats:

- 1/2 a bottle of 75cl white wine

Day 124

Breakfast:

- Cereal and yogurt
- 2 normal crisp breads
- 1 teaspoon of syrup
- 1 peach

Lunch:

- Large bowl of any soup
- 4 crisp breads
- A dish of low fat jelly

Evening meal:

- Medium bowl of chilli
- 1/2 cup of uncooked rice
- Unlimited vegetables

Treats:

- None

Day 125

Breakfast:

- Cereal and yogurt
- 2 crisp breads
- 1/2 a tablespoon of peanut butter
- 1 large orange

Lunch:

- Large bowl of soup
- 2 slices of thick bread

Evening meal:

- 1 large chicken portion
- 1/2 cup of uncooked rice
- Unlimited vegetables

Treats:

- None

Day 126

Breakfast:

- Cereal and yogurt
- 2 crisp breads
- 1 teaspoon of jam
- 1 apple
- 1 orange

Lunch:

- Large bowl of soup
- 2 slices of thick bread

Evening meal:

- 1 medium bowl of homemade stew (any meat)
- 1 cup of uncooked rice
- 1 bowl of low fat jelly

Treats:

- None

Day 127

Weigh day- Stayed the same

Ah well never mind, I have been having a lot of bread lately as I have been very hungry, At least I did not gain, next week should be better as I had hardly any treats last week.

Breakfast:

- Cereal and yogurt
- 2 crisp breads
- 1 tsp of syrup
- 2 pieces of fruit

Lunch:

- 1 large bowl of soup
- 2 thick slices of bread

Evening meal:

- 1 large chicken portion
- 5 small potatoes
- Unlimited vegetables
- 1 tablespoon of mayonnaise

Treats:

- None

Day 128

Breakfast:

- Cereal and yogurt
- 1 piece of fruit
- 2 crisp breads
- 1/2 a teaspoon of syrup

Lunch:

- Large bowl of soup
- 2 slices of thick bread
- Small bowl of Homemade stew (I'm hungry this week)

Evening meal:

- 1/2 of a medium homemade pasty
- 1/2 of a vegetable burger
- 1 cupful of boiled rice
- Unlimited vegetables

Treats:

- 1 measure of brandy

Day 129

Breakfast:

- Cereal and yogurt
- 2 crisp breads
- 1 teaspoon of syrup
- 1 large orange

Lunch:

- Side salad
- 1 large bowl of soup

Evening meal:

- vegetable burger
- 5 small potatoes
- Unlimited vegetables

Treats:

- 2 glasses of wine

Day 130

Breakfast:

- Cereal and yogurt
- 2 crisp breads
- 1 teaspoon of syrup
- 1 large orange

Lunch:

- 1/2 a tin of baked beans
- 2 slices of thick bread
- 2 poached eggs

Evening meal:

- 1 medium bowl of homemade stew
- 1/2 cup of uncooked rice
- Unlimited vegetables

Treats:

- 2 digestive biscuits

Day 131

Breakfast:

- Cereal and yogurt
- 1 large orange
- 2 crisp breads
- 1 teaspoon jam

Lunch:

- Half a pack of noodles cooked any flavor
- 2 slices of thick bread

Evening meal:

- Tuna and salad

Treats:

- 1 bottle of 75cl white wine

Day 132

Breakfast:

- Cereal and yogurt
- 2 crisp breads
- 1 teaspoon of syrup
- 1 piece of any fruit

Lunch:

- 1/2 a pack of noodles cooked
- 2 slices of thick bread

Evening meal:

- 1 medium sausage
- 5 small potatoes
- 1/2 a tin of baked beans
- Unlimited vegetables

Treats:

- 3 brandy measures

Day 133

Breakfast:

- Cereal and yogurt
- 2 crisp breads
- 1/2 a tablespoon of peanut butter
- 1 piece of fruit

Lunch:

- 1 medium bowl of homemade stew

Evening meal:

- 1 vegetable burger
- 5 small potatoes
- Unlimited vegetables

Treats:

- 1/2 a bottle of 75cl white wine
- 1 small brandy

Day 134

Weigh day-2.25 pound (brilliant!) Not only have I lost the 0.25 pound I put on, I also lost an extra 2 pounds as well.

Breakfast:

- Cereal and yogurt
- 2 crisp breads
- 1 teaspoon of jam
- 1 piece of fruit

Lunch:

- 1 medium bowl of stew

Evening meal:

- 1 medium bowl of any meat curry
- 1/2 cup of uncooked rice
- Unlimited vegetables

Treats:

- 1 rum and coke
- 1/2 a bottle of 75cl white wine

Day 135

Breakfast:

- Cereal and yogurt
- 2 crisp breads
- 1/2 a tablespoon of peanut butter
- 1 piece of fruit

Lunch:

- Large bowl of soup
- 4 crisp breads

Evening meal:

- 1 large chicken portion
- 5 small potatoes
- Unlimited vegetables

Treats:

- None

Day 136

Breakfast:

- Cereal and yogurt
- 2 crisp breads
- 1/2 a tablespoon of peanut butter
- 1 piece of fruit

Lunch:

- Large bowl of soup

Evening meal:

- 1 large chicken portion
- 5 small potatoes
- Unlimited vegetables

Treats:

- 1 rum and coke
- 3 glasses of white wine

Day 137

Breakfast:

- Cereal and yogurt
- 1 large rice cake
- 1 teaspoon of jam
- 1 piece of fruit

Lunch:

- 1 large bowl of any soup
- 2 slices of thick bread

Evening meal:

- 1 medium bowl of stew
- 1/2 cup of uncooked rice
- Unlimited vegetables

Treats

- 5 arrow root biscuits

Day 138

Breakfast:

- Cereal and yogurt
- 1 large rice cake
- 1/2 a tablespoon of peanut butter
- 1 piece of fruit

Lunch:

- 1 large bowl of soup

Evening meal:

- 1 large chicken portion
- 5 small potatoes
- Unlimited vegetables

Treats:

- 1/2 a bottle of 75cl white wine
- 2 rice cakes spread with syrup

Day 139

Breakfast:

- Cereal and yogurt
- large rice cake
- 1 teaspoon of syrup
- 2 pieces of fruit

Lunch:

- Large bowl of soup
- 2 slices of thick bread

Evening meal:

- 1 medium bowl of curry
- 1/2 cup of uncooked rice
- Unlimited vegetables

Treats:

- None

Day 140

Breakfast:

- Cereal and yogurt
- 1 large rice cake
- 1/2 a tablespoon of peanut butter
- 1 piece of fruit

Lunch:

- 1 medium bowl of stew
- Side salad

Evening meal:

- 1 medium bowl of curry
- Unlimited vegetables
- no rice

Treats:

- 1/2 a bottle of 75cl white wine

Day 141

Weigh day- 4 pounds!!! wow what a great weight loss, so all together my weight loss is 31.5 ponds and I feel so much better. I have a chance to go out for a meal with friends this week it will be interesting to see what next weeks results will bring. I am now in between 10 a little over 140 pounds my husband reckons I look too thin,

I do believe he is right so I will try and maintain my weight now and probably try and put a bit on. In the next part of my diet I start to add things in, as I have got to where I want to be. The plan now is to stabilize my weight so I can then control it.

Breakfast: (My favorite)

- Cereal and yogurt
- 1 piece of fruit
- 2 crisp breads
- 1 teaspoon of syrup

Lunch:

- 1 large bowl of soup
- 2 slices of thick bread

Evening meal:

- 1 small shank of lamb
- 5 small potatoes

- Unlimited vegetables

Treats:

- 3 digestive biscuits

Day 142

Breakfast:

- Cereal and yogurt
- 2 crisp breads
- 1/2 a tablespoon of peanut butter
- 1 peach
- 1 orange

Lunch:

- 1 medium bowl of curry
- 1/2 cup of uncooked rice

Evening meal:

- 2 slices of thick bread
- 1/2 a tin of beans
- 1 egg

Treats:

- 1/2 a 75cl bottle of white wine
- 1 large piece of cheesecake

Day 143

Breakfast:

- Cereal and yogurt
- 1 apple
- 1 orange
- 2 crisp breads
- 1 teaspoon of syrup

Lunchtime:

- 1 big bowl of soup
- 2 slices of thick bread

Evening meal:

Went out for a 3 course meal by heck I got very full. My stomach must have shrunk. The wine kept flowing too so I have no idea how much of everything that was consumed by me, Time to behave tomorrow I reckon!!!

Treats:

- Everything on offer, ice cream, cream, wine, brandy

Day 144

Breakfast:

- Cereal and yogurt
- 1/2 a tin of fruit salad no juice
- 1 peach
- 2 crisp breads
- 1 teaspoon of syrup

Lunchtime:

- 1 large bowl of soup
- 4 crisp breads

Evening meal:

- 1 8oz steak
- 2 small potatoes
- Unlimited vegetables

Treats:

- 1 glass of wine

Day 145

Breakfast:

- Cereal and yogurt
- 2 crisp breads
- 1/2 a tablespoon of peanut butter
- 1 piece of fruit

Lunch:

- 1/2 a tin of beans
- 2 slices of thick bread
- 2 poached eggs

Evening meal:

- 1 bowl of homemade stew
- Unlimited vegetables

Treats:

- None

Day 146

Breakfast:

- Cereal and yogurt
- 2 crisp breads
- 1/2 a tablespoon of peanut butter
- 1 orange

Lunch:

- 1 big bowl of soup
- 2 slices of thick bread

Evening meal:

- 1 large chicken portion
- 1/2 cup of uncooked rice
- unlimited vegetables

Treats:

- 1 bottle of 75cl white wine
- 1 mars bar

Day 147

Breakfast:

- Cereal and yogurt
- 2 crisp breads
- 1/2 a tablespoon of peanut butter
- peach

Lunch:

- 1 full pack of cooked noodles
- 1 large bowl of soup

Evening meal:

- 1 large piece of fish
- Unlimited vegetables
- 5 small potatoes

Treats:

- 1/2 a liter of dry white wine

Day 148

Weigh day Just as I thought I have stayed the same. Well that's good because in the week I had extra's and went out for a meal. I am increasing the quantity of various foods slightly. 5 gram extra cereal, 1 or 2 ounces extra meat.

Breakfast:

- Cereal and yogurt
- 2 crisp breads
- 1/2 a tablespoon of peanut butter
- 2 pieces of fruit of your choice

Lunch:

- 2 slices of thick bread
- 1/2 a tin of beans
- 2 poached eggs

Evening meal:

- 2 slices of thick bread
- 1 large bowl of soup

Treats:

- 2 large rum and cokes

Day 149

Breakfast:

- Cereal and yogurt
- 2 crisp breads
- 1/2 a tablespoon of peanut butter
- 1 piece of fruit

Lunch:

- 2 slices of thick bread
- 1 large bowl of soup

Evening meal:

- 1 large piece of white fish
- 5 small potatoes
- unlimited vegetables
- 4 tablespoons of parsley sauce

Treats:

Went out for the evening and had
4 large glasses of white wine

Day 150

Breakfast:

- Cereal and yogurt
- 2 crisp breads
- 1 teaspoon of jam
- 1 piece of fruit

Lunch:

- Large bowl of soup
- 2 thick slices of bread

Evening meal:

- 2 vegetable burgers
- 1/2 cup of uncooked rice
- unlimited vegetables

Treats:

- None tonight I have not got any more room left in my tummy. It has definitely shrunk!

Day 151

Breakfast:

- Cereal and yogurt
- 2 crisp breads
- 1/2 a tablespoon of peanut butter
- 1 large piece of fruit

Lunch:

- Tuna and salad
- 2 crisp breads
- 1 peach

Evening meal:

- 1 large chicken portion
- Unlimited vegetables

Treats:

- 4 large glasses of white wine

Day 152

As you are probably aware by now I tend to keep my breakfast pretty much the same as I enjoy it fully, however, I do get fed up sometimes so change it by having two slices of medium sliced bread with either four rashes of any bacon or two sausages cut to fit the bread followed by still having my fruit.

Breakfast:

- Cereal and yogurt
- 2 crisp breads
- 1 teaspoon of honey
- 1 piece of fruit of your choice

Lunch:

- Tuna and salad
- 1 slice of thick bread

Evening meal:

- 1 large pork chop
- Unlimited vegetables
- 5 small potatoes

Treats:

- 1/2 a bottle of 75cl white wine

Day 153

Breakfast:

- Cereal and yogurt
- 2 crisp breads
- 1 apple
- 1/2 an orange
- 1/2 a tablespoon of peanut butter

Lunch:

- Large bowl of soup
- 4 crisp breads

Evening meal:

- 1/2 a tin of beans
- 2 poached eggs
- 2 slices of thick bread

Treats:

- None I am too full again!

Day 154

Breakfast:

- Cereal and yogurt
- 2 crisp breads
- 1/2 a tablespoon of peanut butter
- 1 large piece of fruit

Lunch:

- An 8oz shop bought lasagne
- Unlimited salad

Evening meal:

- 1 large chicken portion
- 5 small potatoes
- Unlimited vegetables

Treats:

- 1/2 a liter of dry white wine

Day 155

Weigh day- 0.75 pound loss. It must be going to the gym that's done it this week. I did go three times mind you. I must not lose any more weight though.

Breakfast:

- 2 slices of thick bread
- 4 rashes of bacon grilled
- 1 poached egg
- 1 orange

Lunch:

- 1 large bowl of soup
- 4 crisp breads

Evening meal:

- Tuna and salad
- 5 small potatoes
- 1 tablespoon of mayonnaise

Treats:

- 1/2 a bottle of 75cl white wine

Day 156

Breakfast:

- Cereal and yogurt
- 2 crisp breads
- 1/2 a tablespoon of peanut butter
- 1 large orange

Lunch:

- Tuna and salad

Evening meal:

- 1 large vegetable burger
- 5 small potatoes
- Unlimited vegetables

Treats:

- 1/2 a bottle of 75cl white wine

Day 157

Breakfast:

- Cereal and yogurt
- 2 crisp breads
- 1/2 a tablespoon of peanut butter
- 1 peach

Lunch:

- 2 slices of thick bread
- 2 poached eggs

Evening meal:

- 1 medium chicken portion
- 1/2 cup of uncooked rice
- Unlimited vegetables

Treats:

- 1/2 a liter of white wine

Day 158

Breakfast:

- Cereal and yogurt
- 2 crisp breads
- 1 teaspoon of honey
- 1 piece of any fruit

Lunch:

- A large bowl of soup
- 4 crisp breads
- Bowl of low fat jelly

Evening meal:

- 1 medium bowl of chilli
- Unlimited vegetables
- No rice

Treats:

- 1/2 a liter of dry white wine

Day 159

Breakfast:

- Cereal and yogurt
- 1 crisp bread
- 2 pieces of fruit
- 1 teaspoon of honey

Lunch:

- 2 poached eggs
- 4 crisp breads

Evening meal:

- Large tin of tuna with salad
- 5 small potatoes
- Unlimited vegetables

Treats:

- 1/2 a liter of dry white wine

Day 160

Breakfast:

- Cereal and yogurt
- 2 crisp breads
- 1 teaspoon of honey
- 1 orange
- 1/2 an apple

Lunch:

- 1 large bowl of soup
- 4 crisp breads

Evening meal:

- 1 large chicken portion
- 5 small potatoes
- Unlimited vegetables

Treats:

- 1 large glass of wine
- 1 mars bar

Day 161

Breakfast:

- Cereal and yogurt
- 2 crisp breads
- 2 teaspoon of jam
- 1 piece of fruit

Lunch:

- 1 slice of thick bread
- 2 poached eggs
- 1 tsp of mayonnaise

Evening meal:

- 1 medium bowl of chilli
- 1/2 cup of uncooked rice
- Unlimited vegetables

Treats:

- 2 glasses of wine
- 1 bag of crisps (any flavor)

Day 162

Weigh day-1 pound loss. Oh dear I had better watch it now as I am starting to look drawn in the face. I think psychologically I am still watching my weight in case I start putting it on. I would stress to anyone who ever follows this way of eating to be careful and eat more to maintain your weight especially if exercising.

Breakfast:

- Cereal and yogurt
- 2 crisp breads
- 1 teaspoon of honey
- 1 peach
- 1 small orange

Lunch:

- 1 vegetable burger
- Side salad

Evening meal:

- 1 large chicken portion
- 5 small potatoes
- Unlimited vegetables
- 3oz of peas

Treats:
- 1/2 a bottle of 75cl white wine

Day 163

Breakfast:

- Cereal and yogurt
- 2 crisp breads
- 1 apple
- 1 orange
- 2 teaspoon of jam

Lunch:

- 1 hard boiled egg
- Side salad
- 2 crisp breads
- 1 tablespoon of mayonnaise

Evening meal:

- 2 large pieces of liver cooked to how you want
- 5 small potatoes
- Unlimited vegetables

Treats:

- 1/2 a liter of white wine

Day 164

Breakfast:

- Cereal and yogurt
- 2 Ryvita fruit crisp breads
- 2 teaspoon of honey
- 1 piece of fruit

Lunch:

- 1 large bowl of soup
- 4 crisp breads

Evening meal:

- Tuna and salad
- 5 small potatoes

Treats:

- 1/2 a liter of dry white wine

Day 165

Breakfast:

- Cereal and yogurt
- 1 large rice cake
- 1 teaspoon of jam

Lunch:

- Went out and had
- Tuna and salad
- One 75cl bottle of white wine

Evening meal:

- 1 medium chicken portion
- 1 cupful of cooked rice
- Unlimited vegetables

Treats:

- None

Day 166

Breakfast:

- Cereal and yogurt
- 2 Ryvita fruit crisp breads
- 2 teaspoon of honey
- 1 peach

Lunch:

- 1 vegetable burger
- Unlimited salad

Evening meal:

- 1 large piece of white fish
- 5 small potatoes
- Unlimited vegetables
- 2 crisp breads

Treats:

- 1/2 a bottle of 75cl white wine

Day 167

Breakfast:

- Cereal and yogurt
- 2 crisp breads
- 2 teaspoon of jam
- 1 peach

Lunch:

- 1 large piece of white fish
- 4 Ryvita crisp breads

Evening meal:

- 1 large chicken portion
- 1/2 cup of uncooked rice
- Unlimited vegetables

Treats:

- 1 glass of wine
- 1 apple

Day 169

Breakfast:

- Cereal and yogurt
- 2 Ryvita fruit crisp breads
- 2 teaspoon of jam
- 1 peach

Lunch:

- 1 large bowl of soup
- 4 crisp breads

Evening meal:

- 1/2 a tin of baked beans
- 2 poached eggs
- 4 crisp breads

Treats:

- 1/2 a liter of dry white wine
- 1 small packet of Maltesers

Day 170

Weigh day, Stayed the same today it must be the extra chocolate that I had that maintained the weight because the food is pretty much the same

Breakfast:

- Cereal and yogurt
- 2 Ryvita fruit crisp breads
- 2 teaspoon of syrup
- 1 peach

Lunch:

- 1 large bowl of soup
- 2 slices of thick bread

Evening meal:

- 1 medium bowl of curry
- 1/2 cup of uncooked rice
- Medium pile of cooked green beans

Treats:

- 1/2 a bottle of 75cl white wine
- 1 mars bar

Day 171

Breakfast:

- Cereal and yogurt
- 2 Ryvita fruit crisp breads
- 2 teaspoon of jam
- 1 orange

Lunch:

- 1 medium bowl of cooked pasta mixed with a tin of tuna
- 1 tablespoon of mayonnaise

Evening meal:

- 1 medium bowl of Bolognaise
- 1 cupful of cooked pasta

Treats:

- None

Day 172

Breakfast:

- Cereal and yogurt
- 2 normal crisp breads
- 2 teaspoon of syrup
- 1 peach

Lunch:

- 2 poached eggs
- 1/2 a tin of baked beans
- 4 crisp breads

Evening meal:

- 1 large chicken portion
- 5 small potatoes
- Unlimited vegetables

Treats:

- 1 peach
- 2 glasses of white wine

Day 173

Breakfast:

- Cereal and yogurt
- 1 large rice cake
- 1 teaspoon of syrup
- 1 peach
- 1 small orange

Lunch:

- 1 medium piece of fish
- Unlimited salad

Evening meal:

- 2 vegetable burgers
- 1/2 cup of uncooked rice
- Unlimited vegetables

Treats:

- 1/2 a bottle of 75cl white wine

Day 174

Breakfast:

- Cereal and yogurt
- 2 crisp breads
- 2 teaspoon of jam
- 1 peach
- 1 small orange

Lunch:

- Large bowl of soup
- 4 crisp breads

Evening meal:

- 1 large chicken portion
- 5 small potatoes
- unlimited vegetables

Treats:

- Went out later and had a pizza (oops)

Day 175

Breakfast:

- Cereal and yogurt
- 2 crisp breads
- 2 teaspoon of syrup
- 1 peach
- 1 small orange

Lunch:

- 1/2 a tin of baked beans
- 2 poached eggs
- 4 crisp breads

Remember with this one, I lay the crisp breads on a plate, pour the beans on top of them followed by the poached eggs. ummmm yummy!

Evening meal:

- 1 Medium piece of fish
- Unlimited vegetables

Treats:

- 1/2 a bottle of 75cl white wine

Day 176

Breakfast:

- Cereal and yogurt
- 2 crisp breads
- 2 teaspoon of syrup
- 1 peach
- 1 small orange

Lunch:

- 1/4 of a homemade pizza
- Unlimited salad

Evening meal:

- 1 medium pork chop
- Unlimited vegetables

Treats:

- 1 bottle of 75cl white wine

Day 177

Weigh day+1   I have gained this week which is good for me at this point so if I still wanted to carry on losing the weight I would leave out things like the pizza and cut down on the wine the rest is pretty much the same. I am finally in control.

Breakfast:

- Cereal and yogurt
- 2 crisp breads
- 2 teaspoon of syrup
- 1 peach
- 1 orange

Lunch:

- 1 hard boiled egg
- Unlimited salad
- 1 tablespoon of mayonnaise
- 4 crisp breads

Evening meal:

- 1 medium chicken portion
- Unlimited vegetables

Treats:

- 1/2 a liter of white wine

Day 178

Breakfast

- Cereal and yogurt
- 1 large rice cake
- 1 crisp bread
- 2 teaspoon of syrup
- 1 peach
- 1 small orange

Lunch:

- 1 large bowl of soup
- 2 large rice cakes

Evening meal:

- 1 medium bowl of curry
- 1/2 cup of uncooked rice
- Unlimited vegetables

Treats:

- 1/2 a liter of white wine

Day 179

Breakfast:

- Cereal and yogurt
- 1 large rice cake
- 1 teaspoon of jam
- 1 peach
- 1 orange

Lunch:

- 1 large bowl of soup
- 2 slices of thick bread

Evening meal:

- Medium chicken portion
- 5 small potatoes
- Unlimited vegetables

Treats:

- 1/2 a 75cl bottle of white wine

Day 180

Breakfast:

- Cereal and yogurt
- 1 large rice cake
- 1 teaspoon of syrup
- 1 peach
- 1 orange

Lunch:

- 2 slices of thick bread
- 1/2 a tin of baked beans
- 2 poached eggs

Evening meal:

- Medium chicken portion
- 5 small potatoes
- Unlimited vegetables

Treats:

- 1/2 a bottle of 75cl white wine
- 1 mars bar

Day 181

Breakfast:

- Cereal and yogurt
- 1 large rice cake
- 1 teaspoon of jam
- 1 orange

Lunch:

- 1 pack of flavored noodles cooked

Evening meal:

- 1 large piece of chicken
- Unlimited vegetables

Treats:

- 1/2 a bottle of 75cl white wine
- 1 glass of cider

Day 182

Breakfast:

- Cereal and yogurt
- 1 large rice cake
- 1 peach

Lunch:

- 1 large bowl of soup
- 2 slices of thick bread

Evening meal:

- Medium portion of spaghetti carbonara
- Salad

Treats:

- 1/2 a bottle of 75cl white wine
- 1 glass of cider

Day 183

Breakfast:

- Cereal and yogurt
- 2 crisp breads
- 1 teaspoon of jam
- 1 peach

Lunch:

- 1 Cupful of cooked pasta
- Unlimited salad
- 1 large dish of jelly

Evening meal:

- 1 large chicken portion
- 4 small potatoes
- Unlimited vegetables

Treats:

- 1/2 a 75cl bottle of white wine

Day 184

Weigh day Final. My weight has maintained itself this week so I am pretty much in control of it now, if I go up I just leave some things out of it for one week and if I go down I increase my treats. I love this way of eating I think it would work for most people. Not everyone would like to have chicken so often so the meat preference could be changed. I chose chicken because I like it and I can have a lot of it. I could have chosen red meat and had a little less of it.

Breakfast:

- Cereal and yogurt
- 2 crisp breads
- 2 teaspoon of syrup
- 1 piece of fruit

Lunch:

- 1 large bowl of soup
- 2 thick slices of bread

Evening meal:

- 1 large chicken portion
- 5 small potatoes
- Unlimited vegetables

Treats:

- None. Going out for a meal in a couple of days

Day 185

Breakfast:

- Cereal and yogurt
- 2 crisp breads
- 1 teaspoon of jam
- 1 peach

Lunch:

- 1 large bowl of soup
- 4 crisp breads

Evening meal:

- 1 large chicken portion
- 5 small potatoes
- Unlimited vegetables

Treats:

- None

Today is the final day of the six months, and tonight I am going out to dinner. I have got this far, and I am where I want to be with my weight. I suppose I should congratulate myself.

I am not going to write anything down today I want a day where I can have whatever I want then just to keep an eye on it as from tomorrow. I intend to weigh once a week and adjust my food accordingly.

I have learned that I need to adjust my food slightly rather than drastically to suit my weight gain or loss and to wait for results. Weighing each week will allow me to regulate my weight before it becomes an issue. In the past I had put, 10 pounds on before I realized I had a problem. Then I had the crash diet syndrome to get it off. I have written this book six months after finishing the initial six months of dieting. My weight has remained within 3 pounds up and down throughout the past few months and even over Christmas 2013. I have only gained 4 extra pounds and have already lost 1.5 of those pounds.

Enjoy your food and your wine and be happy.

Other Titles by Jackie Clark:

Quick and Easy Recipes Baking
Quick and Easy Recipes Hot & Spicy
Quick and Easy Recipes Pasties Bakes Boats
Quick and Easy Recipes Savoury
Quick and Easy Recipes Barbeque and Garlic
Quick and Easy Recipes Sauces
Quick and Easy Recipes Pancakes
Quick and Easy Recipes Favourites
Quick and Easy Recipes Whole Collection 1
Quick and Easy Recipes Whole Collection 2
Baking The Cake

Join Jackie's web site to gain access to free recipes.

Helpful cooking information and be kept up to date of any new titles as they become available. These are usually at a discount for site members.

http://jackieclark.ebookvillage.co.uk